GUT FIRST, SCIENCE SECOND

Health Consequences of the Trump Doctrine

A

PATRIOTIC

PAMPHLET

BY

Andrew Goldstein

(sixoneseven) Books
Boston, Massachusetts 2020

Permissions requests may be addressed to:

SixOneSeven Books
P.O. Box 1391
Concord, MA 01742
www.sixonesevenbooks.com

Cover design by Max Goldstein. Interior by Eliyanna Kaiser.

Boston / Andrew Goldstein—First Edition
ISBN 978-0-9848245-6-4

Printed in the United States of America

We have it in our power to begin the world over again.

THOMAS PAINE

Author's Note

I'M NOT A SCIENTIST OR PROFESSOR OR politician or an expert. I'm not famous. I am simply a 72-year-old citizen of the United States who believes that the next presidential election will be the most important one in my lifetime. If you are an independent voter or a moderate Republican or a wavering Democrat, then I'm hoping that you will read my pamphlet.

Our children and grandchildren are depending on us to provide them a healthy future, but President Trump's environmental policies are endangering their lives. Our families are becoming casualties of two of the main tenets of Trump's environmental agenda: 1) Gut first, Science second; and 2) Corporations over People.

I play in a weekly poker game—currently suspended by the virus—with mostly Trump supporters. We've learned not to talk politics because we're simply unable to have a rational discussion. I can't believe they believe the lies and distortions President Trump tells, and they can't believe that I don't see the mainstream press, the New York Times, CNN, NPR, et al, as fake news. Luckily, politics isn't the reason we get together. We enjoy each other's company, the gambling, and the excitement of a new world being created with every shuffle.

As a nation, however, we don't have the luxury of avoiding the political discussion: The stakes are too high. Because many of the worst consequences of Trump's policies will occur decades from now, it's sometimes hard to grasp the full extent of the damage he is doing, but our recent experience with the coronavirus teaches us that we need to address problems before they grow to huge and life- threatening magnitude. The virus also shows us how quickly the world can change. We take our beautiful planet for granted. As Americans we assume life will continue as we know it and that we are the masters of the universe. We are not. Even with our nuclear weapons and high-tech marvels like artificial intelligence, we are fragile. A microscopic bug can bring the most powerful country in the world to its knees. The booming world we thought was permanent and structurally sound has been exposed as vulnerable. Suddenly things are not so good. Free and happy lifestyles succumb to lockdowns. The economy goes from robust to anemic. Millions of workers lose their jobs. Many people become deathly ill. Hospitals can barely keep up. The death toll mounts. And this all happens in a matter of months. The world is upended.

President Trump's leadership on the virus has been disastrous, but on the environment he's even worse because he's actively pursuing policies that will harm us all instead of making choices for our health and the health of the planet. He has consistently prioritized corporations over people. Some may think it's hyperbole to say that President Trump's corporations-first agenda has evolved into a war against the environment, with science taking a back seat, and children becoming collateral damage. You may think I am exaggerating when I say that he has set time-bombs that are going to inflict harm on future generations. You may think that anything written that is critical of him is political in nature or, worse yet, fake news. But you can easily research and verify every assertion in this pamphlet.

In my view, those of us lucky enough to have been born in the United States or to have immigrated here should awake every morning and give thanks for the incredible bounty of resources bestowed on us. Rich soil and fresh water, rivers and two oceans, flora, mountains and lakes, gorgeous vistas and wildlife. To be alive in what in many ways is a paradise is to be blessed.

Whether you believe you earned this bounty or it was given to you by God or good karma from past lives or the luck of the draw, I think many of us can agree that there should be a simple unwritten contract which states: *We may share in the bounty that is the natural world of the United States and all that is asked of us that we don't harm it. Ideally, on our way out we leave it better than when we entered, but at the very least we don't make it worse.*

President Trump has launched a barrage of rulings that favor the profitability of corporations at the expense of children and the environment. He is poisoning our air and water, resulting in collateral damage not only to children and the environment but to senior citizens and other vulnerable populations.

There is no original research in this pamphlet. The facts have already been published in government records, scientific journals, magazine articles, and newspapers. However, with all the noise and other controversies, many of the facts have been drowned out and obscured. I have tried to expose the damage that President Trump has caused, by laying out the facts clearly and honestly and with ample documentation. I hope you will read the pamphlet with an open mind and then ask yourself if you can, in good conscience, accept what's happening to the country we will leave to our children.

Introduction

———————————————

PRESIDENT TRUMP'S MISHANDLING OF the COVID-19 crisis graphically illustrates the dire consequences of his approach to scientific issues. His strong inclination is to "go with his gut" rather than listen to scientists and experts. Making decisions from his gut might sometimes work in real estate (though various Trump enterprises have gone bankrupt a half-dozen times), but if his gut leads him to ignore scientific reality in making public health decisions, tens of thousands of people could die unnecessarily, hundreds of thousands more could fall seriously ill, and millions could lose their jobs.

This is as true with the climate crisis as it is with the pandemic. And unfortunately, this same modus operandi is at the core of his environmental policy. If we don't recognize the flaws in his approach, the damage this pandemic has caused to our health and our economy could easily be dwarfed by future environmental catastrophes.

In that way, the pandemic serves as a warning of what happens when a president disregards scientific advice in the belief that he knows better and thus fails to act at a critical time when bold, decisive actions could make a difference. On President Trump's watch, we are currently in the worst peacetime health crisis in the United States in over 100 years and the worst economic crisis since the Great Depression.

Two hundred and fifteen countries have been infected by the COVID-19 virus, but the United States has more virus-related deaths than any other country. We also have more virus-related deaths per million of population than 206 countries, which puts us at the bottom tier of protecting citizens from the pandemic, in 207th place.[i]

Compare the United States' record with that of countries acting promptly on the advice of their scientists. South Korea, Vietnam, Germany, Iceland, Israel, and New Zealand competently controlled the virus, resulting in fewer deaths and less economic upheaval. Admittedly, every country is unique, with its own political systems, cultures, values, and population densities. It is not totally fair to compare one country's results with another, but the United States has done so poorly compared with almost every country in the world that at some point the excuses become lame. South Korea had its first reported case of the virus on January 19, the same day the first documented case was reported in the United States. The former nation immediately started large-scale testing, contact tracing, and quarantining. During the next eight-week period, from January 19 to March 15, when South Korea was defending itself, the United States did little beyond imposing a couple of partial travel bans to contain the spread of the virus. As of July 1, 2020, South Korea had 282 coronavirus deaths, and six deaths per million of population. As of the same date, the United States had 130,446 coronavirus deaths and 394 deaths per million of population, almost 66 times more deaths per million than South Korea had. If the US had done as effective a job as South Korea, we would have had only 1,986 deaths.[ii] Maybe with our individualistic culture and political structure, we couldn't have done as well as South Korea. But if we had a president who knew how to lead during a crisis, we certainly could have reduced the number of American deaths.

In this pandemic, the most serious health consequences of the Trump approach have mainly hit the elderly and essential workers. However, the health consequences of his gut-centered and corporations-first approach to environmental issues will primarily affect our children and grandchildren. They will be the collateral damage of the Trump agenda.

COVID-19 has shouted out its warning. We must listen.

The Environment

———————

—COAL—

COAL IS A DYING INDUSTRY, which is good for the natural world but not good for people who earn their living mining coal. In the 1920's almost a million Americans mined coal. Today, only 50,000 coal miners are still operating in the United States. A humane government would invest in these people, training them for new industries such as solar and wind power. Retraining these miners not only would give them a new way of making a living; it would also protect their health, since more than 10 percent of coal miners with more than 25 years of experience end up with black lung disease.[iii]

On February 16, 2017, less than one month into his presidency, Trump repealed the Stream Protection Rule, which had limited coal companies' ability to dump coal-mining waste into rivers and streams. Coal companies are now freer to pollute our waterways.

The Stream Protection Rule was intended to reduce "acid mine runoff." Water becomes more acidic when there is a chemical reaction between water and rocks, such as coal, that contain sulfur-bearing minerals, resulting in sulfuric acid. This acid then leaches heavy metals out of rocks, creating toxic fluids that can harm plants, animals, and humans.[iv]

To be fair, this elimination of the Stream Protection Rule wasn't only Trump's doing. We also have Mitch McConnell leading the way in the Senate. McConnell, from the coal state of Kentucky, doesn't seem to care much about the health of his constituents. Consider: US Representative John Yarmuth also from Kentucky, opposed the rule's repeal. He contended that the Stream Protection Rule was "one of the only safety measures that would protect these families from poisoned drinking water, higher rates of cancer, lung disease, respiratory illness, cardiovascular disease, birth defects and the countless negative health effects that plague this region."

Yarmuth brought polluted well water from a constituent's home in Pike County to Washington and challenged his Republican colleagues to drink it, saying he would vote to repeal the Stream Protection Rule if one of them was brave enough to swallow the water. None of his fellow lawmakers accepted the challenge.[v]

Think about that for a moment. The Republican lawmakers refused to drink the water, yet Trump and those lawmakers had no qualms about repealing the Stream Protection Rule, which meant that polluted and poisoned water would be streaming into the homes of American citizens, who are less powerful and protected than their legislators.

The justification is deregulation; the reduction or elimination of regulations in a particular industry. In theory, this might have economic benefits, but they must be weighed against the dangers of unregulated businesses. What is the acceptable collateral damage of deregulation in the coal industry? Clearly, any harm to the lawmakers wasn't acceptable but harm to families living near toxic waterways was. How many poisonings are okay? How many deaths are okay? A hundred, a thousand? Ten thousand? A study in the Journal of American Medical Association (JAMA), based on data from the Environmental Protection Agency (EPA), concluded that 80,000 deaths and more than one million people with respiratory problems every decade would be collateral damage from Trump's consistently anti-environmental agenda.[vi]

Let's say the data or the conclusions are exaggerated and only 40,000 people will die and only half a million people will get sick with respiratory problems. Or cut that in half or in half again. At what point do you say that it's okay for only 20,000 or 10,000 Americans to die so mining companies can make higher profits by poisoning our streams? Common sense would simply say, "No, you can't harm American families by dumping poison into our waterways." Lawmakers who cared about our country and its people would say, "If water is not good enough for me to drink, then it's not good enough for the average citizen."

Why introduce legislation that is going to create health problems and cause avoidable deaths? By what calculus does that make sense? We know that President Trump appointed a former coal lobbyist to be the head of the EPA. We know that fossil fuel companies, including coal companies like Murray Energy, gave millions of dollars to

Trump's inauguration festivities.[vii] While we can't be sure of Trump's motives, we do know that prioritizing corporations over the health of people has been a consistent theme throughout his presidency.

Over and over again, Trump has made or changed rules that help corporations, while inflicting harm on people and the environment. In 2018, the Trump administration suspended the Steam Electric Power Generating Effluent Guidelines, which required coal-fired power plants to treat toxics in the wastewater they discharge. The Trump administration proposed a much more anemic rule instead, which has resulted in the yearly discharge into nearby rivers of over one billion pounds of pollutants, including toxic levels of mercury, arsenic, lead, and selenium.[viii]

THE BURNING OF COAL POLLUTES OUR environment, leaving tiny particles of soot in the air that increase the likelihood of respiratory diseases such as asthma, cancer, and heart dysfunctions. It also fuels global warming and contributes to the buildup of mercury in our atmosphere. According to the World Health Organization, "Mercury is highly toxic to human health, posing a particular threat to the development of the child."[ix] It damages the brains of fetuses and babies and increases the likelihood of heart attacks in adults. Neurological symptoms of mercury poisoning include mental retardation, seizures, vision and hearing impairment, and memory loss.[x] There is no known safe level of exposure.

On April 16, 2020, with the coronavirus killing on average over 2,000 Americans a day and evidence mounting that coronavirus patients who have asthma or live in areas with high levels of air pollution are more likely to die, the Trump administration finalized a major change in how the government quantifies the dangers of air pollution. Under Trump's revisions to the Mercury and Air Toxics Standards, government scientists will no longer be able to count the reduction of smog and soot as a benefit of regulating power plants. Though this new rule doesn't increase the amount of mercury allowed, it makes it much more difficult to decrease it. The Trump government is governing on the principle that it's not necessary to reduce mercury and other harmful pollutants from power plants. The new rule, by default, will allow more soot and air pollutants, more mercury, more asthma and respiratory illnesses, more harm to children, and more premature deaths.[xi]

Along with other matters of racial disparity that are now taking center stage, this ruling will particularly have adverse effects on minority communities. As we have seen with the coronavirus, Black, Latinx, and Native Americans are dying at higher rates than white Americans. Many factors are involved, but underlying health issues such as high rates of asthma and living in more polluted environments appear to make these populations especially vulnerable to the virus.[xii]

—CHLORPYRIFOS—

CHLORPYRIFOS, A DOW CHEMICAL PRODUCT is another compound where the label No Known Safe Level of Exposure should be stamped on its packaging. Chlorpyrifos is a neurotoxic pesticide sprayed on corn, wheat, apples, broccoli, oranges, and many other fruits and vegetables. It has been found to harm wildlife, is extremely toxic, and is particularly harmful to children, causing many developmental problems, including attention disorders, delayed motor development, memory issues, and low IQs. In more severe cases it can also cause convulsions, respiratory paralysis, and death.[xiii]

In 1996 the United States Congress unanimously passed The Food Quality Protection Act, which allows a pesticide to be used only if there is "a reasonable certainty of no harm." In 2016, after years of study, the EPA recommended banning Chlorpyrifos. According to Earthjustice, the EPA found that:

- "All food exposures exceed safe levels, with children ages one to two exposed to levels of Chlorpyrifos that are 140 times what EPA deems safe."

- "There is no safe level of Chlorpyrifos in drinking water."[xiv]

A noncontroversial, nonpartisan, common sense ban on Chlorpyrifos should have been enacted. The ban was also recommended by the American Academy of Pediatrics. However, Donald J. Trump became president, and his EPA reversed its intention to ban Chlorpyrifos.

Dow Chemical gave one million dollars to Trump's inauguration fund.[xv]

— C LEAN P OWER P LAN —

PRESIDENT TRUMP HAS REVERSED OR proposed to reverse almost 100 hundred environmental rules. He's poisoning the air we breathe and water we drink, and he's fueling global warming. A prime example is his repeal of the Clean Power Plan. This plan is a provision under the Clean Air Act, our country's main law controlling air pollution. The Clean Power Plan would reduce carbon emissions from power plants and decrease the air pollution, which contributes to many respiratory diseases, both helping in the fight against global warming and making air safer for future generations. "In 2030 alone, there would be 870 million fewer tons of carbon pollution. This is like canceling out the annual carbon emissions from 70 percent of the nation's cars or avoiding the pollution from the yearly electricity use of every home in America." [xvi]

In 2015, President Obama's EPA estimated the Clean Power Plan could prevent, annually, between 1,500 to 3,600 premature deaths. In 2017, President Trump's EPA estimated the Clean Power Plan could prevent up to 4,500 premature deaths annually as well as 90,000 asthma attacks in children over a decade.

President Trump ignored his scientist's warnings and repealed the Clean Power Plan. (Like some of the other Trump proposals and repeals, the repeal of the Clean Power Plan is being fought in our courts.) In 2018, two Harvard university researchers concluded that repealing the rule would lead to an estimated 36,000 deaths and nearly 630,000 cases of respiratory infection in children over a decade. [xvii] Regardless of which estimates are correct, the results are disease and death to children in the United States.

Repealing the Clean Power Plan is part of a month by month prolonged attack against all of us. It's a systematic weakening of the immune system of our country. Before

Trump started attacking the structures that have been improving air quality, pollution had been decreasing. Under Trump's leadership, air pollution began increasing, only temporarily slowed because of the constraints of the pandemic. Carbon dioxide levels just set a record high in May 2020, probably the highest it has been in three million years.[xviii] To combat this increase, Trump didn't rescind any of his anti-environmental measures or introduce new tougher legislation to reduce air pollution. Instead, in May 2019, his administration announced plans to change the way the EPA calculates the health risks of air pollution. As a result, they have been able to report fewer deaths caused by pollution.[xix] It's a clever tactic. The administration makes and changes rules that increase pollution and then changes the rules that calculate the impact of that pollution as well as limiting which scientific studies are allowed to be used in the calculations.

So, this three-prong attack of changing the rules to allow more air pollution, altering the metrics by which the health risks of air pollution are measured, and banning certain scientific studies, combine to create a more toxic environment for children both now and in the future. This toxicity also makes the elderly more vulnerable when a virus such as COVID-19 invades our country.

— TIME BOMBS —

HERE ARE FIVE OTHER TIME-BOMBS President Trump has set. (Google The Trump Administration Is Reversing 100 Environmental rules to see the full list.) Whether you're a Trump supporter or never-Trumper or an undecided voter, ask yourself whether these policies are good for the health of your family and all the living species on the planet, or are they mainly good for oil, gas, coal, and chemical companies?

- He canceled a requirement for oil and gas companies to report methane emissions and proposed to remove methane transmission and storage from regulation. Methane is a powerful greenhouse gas that contributes to climate change. This proposal will result in more frequent and serious asthma attacks as well as heart disease.[xx]

- He withdrew a proposed rule aimed at reducing pollutants in the air and at sewage treatment plants. Combined with rejecting EPA scientists' recommendations to strengthen the standard restricting fine particles in the air, this action will lead to thousands of premature deaths of individuals sensitive to air pollution.[xxi]

- He proposed a rule exempting certain types of power plants from parts of an EPA rule limiting toxic discharges from power plants into public waterways.[xxii]

- He revoked California's power to set its own more stringent emissions standards for cars and light trucks as well as, in a separate ruling, rolling back clean car regulation and fuel economy standards for the entire country. By 2050, this rule will translate into 18,500 premature deaths due largely to higher levels of small particles in the air.[xxiii]

• In January of 2020, he replaced the Waters of the United States Rule with the Navigable Waters Protection Rule. This new rule rolls back many of the protections from polluters to wetlands and streams that had been in effect since 1972 under the Clean Water Act, which was signed by Republican President Nixon. It also frees landowners to pollute without getting permits. "This will be the biggest loss of clean water protection the country has ever seen," said Blan Holman, a lawyer specializing in federal water policy at the Southern Environmental Law Center. Should you be skeptical of bias from an environmental law center, consider that the EPA's Scientific Advisory Board of 41 government scientists, many appointed by the Trump administration, concluded that the new Trump water rule ignores science by "failing to acknowledge watershed systems. They found 'no scientific justification' for excluding certain bodies of water from protection under the new regulations."[xxiv]

Stop for a second and think about this: The EPA's Scientific Advisory Board, including mainly Trump appointees, said the revised changes to the Waters of the United States Rule "decreases protection for our nation's waters and does not support the objective of restoring and maintaining 'the chemical, physical and biological integrity' of these waters." Not the Democrats, not Obama appointees, not the fake news media, not Nancy Pelosi, not the Deep State, but scientists who Trump himself chose are telling him that weakening of the Waters of the United States Rule is a bad idea.

According to scientists and data from the EPA, President Trump's environmental policies will end up killing more Americans than all of the mass shooters in the history of our country combined, as well as more Americans than died in the wars in Korea, Iraq, Afghanistan, and Vietnam. A similar statement can be made about the death toll caused by President Trump's mishandling of the coronavirus. His gut first, science second approach to public health policy threatens the well-being of all Americans.

Climate Change

—FACTS—

THROUGHOUT THE WORLD, PEOPLE are going to starve, migrate and die from climate-related events such as floods, fires, droughts, and from diseases caused by migrating insects and contaminated water. In 2014 the World Health Organization predicted on average 250,000 deaths a year between 2030-2050 because of climate change. More recent studies are predicting over 500,000 climate related deaths by 2050.[xxv] While skeptics may dismiss these warnings as "the sky is falling" hysteria, many others believe that the threat from climate change is actually much worse and the actual deaths will be higher than predicted.

Scientists believe that in addition to bringing severe storms, flooding, and droughts, climate change will adversely affect water sources throughout the world, in turn affecting our food supply, health, industry, ecosystems, and transportation. It will cause more pollution and more diseases, heat waves, stronger hurricanes, higher sea levels, and an Arctic free of ice.[xxvi] More animals will become extinct due to loss of habitat. Agriculture will suffer from increased diversity of pests, loss of arable land, crop failures, and livestock shortages. "The American Medical Association has reported an increase in mosquito-borne diseases like malaria and dengue fever, as well as a rise in cases of chronic conditions like asthma, most likely as a direct result of global warming."[xxvii]

Most people in the United States now accept the reality of climate change. I want to emphasize the following reasons why they do.

- The last ten years are the warmest the oceans have been in our recorded history.[xxviii]

- In 2019 the World Meteorological Association confirmed that not only were the previous four years the warmest on record on land, but 20 of the last 22 years were the warmest ever recorded.[xxix]

- Ice is melting in the Arctic Circle and in Antarctica.[xxx]

- According to NASA's satellite data, glaciers are retreating in the Alps, Himalayas, Andes, Rockies, Alaska, and Africa.[xxxi]

- Sea levels are rising, coastlines are shrinking.[xxxii]

- Coral reefs in the Florida Keys and the Great Barrier Reef in Australia have been shrinking for decades. Arctic animals are declining. The permafrost is melting rapidly in the Arctic, Siberia, and the Himalayas. Around the world, mountain snowpack is declining. Droughts are becoming more frequent and torrential rains and flooding are increasing.[xxxiii]

The debate is over. Climate change is happening. There are no alternative facts. There may be alternative opinions on the causes of climate change and the severity of the consequences, but the change is happening, and it is only going to get worse.

—President Trump and Climate Change—

CLIMATE CHANGE BEGAN BEFORE TRUMP and will be a serious problem long after he's gone. He's not the first president to fail to address it. However, he is the first president to aggressively enact laws that make the problem worse. His environmental agenda increases air pollution and toxic water. It allows more CO_2 and methane in the atmosphere, which almost all climate scientists believe contributes to the unprecedented speed of climate change. The only remaining debate, and I use the word loosely, is whether human activity is causing the changes. Ninety-seven percent of climate scientists throughout the world believe that fossil fuel use is driving the climate changes. Some 197 international scientific organizations now believe that global warming is real and has been caused by human action.[xxxiv]

Years ago, even when almost every study showed that cigarette smoking was a main cause of lung cancer, there were always a few skeptics who published other theories.

Waiting for 100 percent agreement, no matter how much evidence is produced, is a futile exercise. We know climate change is happening and almost all climate scientists believe fossil fuels are the main culprit.

Many departments in the federal government, such as Homeland Security, Department of Defense, Department of Agriculture, Department of Commerce, the intelligence agencies, the military, and NASA take the threat of global warming seriously and have plans to deal with it.[xxxv] President Trump and his fossil-fuel allies in Congress ignore the advice from scientists.

Over the years, Trump has made conflicting statements about climate change. Some are ridiculous: "The concept of global warming was created by and for the Chinese in order to make U.S. manufacturing non-competitive." Some are conspiratorial: "The weather has been so cold for so long that the global warming HOAXSTERS had to change the name to climate change." Others acknowledge the problem but deny the cause: "I don't think it's a hoax, I think there's probably a difference. But I don't know that it's man made."[xxxvi]

According to the Sabin Center for Climate Change Law, the Trump administration has taken more than 130 steps to scale back measures to fight climate change. Withdrawing from the Paris Climate Agreement, lifting the ban on drilling in the arctic National Wildlife Refuge, opening up nine million acres of Western land to oil and gas drilling, and proposing to eliminate restrictions that require newly built coal power plants to capture carbon dioxide emissions are just a few of those actions.[xxxvii]

On March 31, 2020, President Trump announced his "final rule to roll-back Obama-era automobile fuel efficiency standards, relaxing efforts to limit climate-warming tailpipe pollution and virtually undoing the government's biggest effort to combat climate change."[xxxviii] This new rule would allow over a billion tons more carbon dioxide into the air. The government scientists, many appointed by President Trump, concluded that there were significant weaknesses in the scientific analysis of Trump's new rule.[xxxix]

As he has done many times before, Trump disregarded the finding of scientists. No wonder that Christine Whitman, the former Republican governor of New Jersey and the administrator of the EPA under George W. Bush, said, "It's been a war on science since Trump came in." Or that Presidential historian David Brinkley said, "Donald Trump is the most anti-science and anti-environment president we've ever had." Or that Columbia University has tracked more than 200 examples of Trump's administration's attempts to limit scientific research or the use of scientific information in some way.[xl]

In 2018, scientists and agencies in the Trump government issued a report stating that unchecked global warming could both cost the United States hundreds of billions of dollars annually and damage the health of all of us. This wasn't Barack Obama or Hillary Clinton or the Democrats in Congress issuing a warning. This was the warning and conclusion from the scientists working for President Trump. His response: "I don't believe it."[xli]

Scientists throughout the world have been shouting warnings for decades. They are prescribing remedies and solutions to deal with climate change. The time has come to take action before events spiral out of control. We are at that urgent inflection point. Scientists say we need to act boldly on climate change in the next ten years or risk irreversible catastrophic consequences.

The creatures of our world, including your children and grandchildren, are depending on you to think this through carefully. Do you really want someone who has shown little regard for our health and is ignoring scientific evidence to lead our country for another four years?

"Fore"

———————

–WATCH OUT–

IN THE TRUMP DOCTRINE THERE ARE
those two intertwined and twisted hierarchies: 1) gut first,
science second and 2) corporations over people. Both of
these hierarchies are damaging our health and the environment. COVID-19 has shouted out its warning. We've
now seen firsthand how chaotic and destructive Trump's
approach to the virus has been. A major lesson from
COVID-19 is that, in the time of a pandemic, science is
important. This is even more true when dealing with the
environment. Don't we want a President who understands
the health consequences of dumping poisons into our
air and water, a President who listens to scientists when
they tell him that his policies are going to sicken and kill
children?

To maintain our health, lifestyle, and economy, we

need a President who believes in science, believes in climate change, and is passionate about aggressively leading the world in trying to fix it.

— A Way Out—

THE CORONAVIRUS PANDEMIC HELPS US break through the fog to see clearly what is important: our family, our friends, our health, our country, our work, caring for others, and being alive. For the religious: our God. It helps us to see what is noble: the health care workers, the first responders, the people who are willing to sacrifice their health to care for us. It doesn't matter whether they are liberal or conservative or white or black or Latinx or Asian or Native American.

The virus doesn't care whether you are a Democrat or Republican or Independent. We need to find a way to overcome these divisions to protect our earth, our air, our water, our climate, life as we know it. The time has come to nurture this gift of life on Earth. We are the living, the breathing, the sentient stewards, and we owe it to our children and grandchildren to pass on the bounty of a healthy biosphere. We owe it to them to leave this wonder, this Earth, alive and thriving, not choking and dying like bleached coral reefs.

The bounty that is life, the natural world, the miracle that is our Earth, the stunning array of creatures and flowers and trees and landscapes, the sheer wonder of breath, of thought, of movement, and sight and sound and taste and touch and smell. Pause and think about it, how lucky we are, how fortunate. Life. Breath. The gift.

The Earth too wants to breathe. Let's lead the world in climate repair. Let's join forces with other countries and start a Manhattan project together, not to be the first to build an atomic weapon, but to build as a whole community, a whole earth, the new technologies, the new shields, the new fabric of a society less dependent on fossil fuels and more determined to preserve and care for our planet. Let's show the next generation and the one after it that in 2020 the people of the United States, regardless of their political differences, banded together as a country to protect the amazing planet Earth and the gift of breath.

This may sound naïve, but past generations of Americans created a democracy, ended slavery, helped save the world from Nazism, and put a man on the moon. It's now our time for the next great feat. Let's vote in November for science, our children, and for all the creatures of the world. Let's join forces under the banner of a great purpose: showing gratitude to God or the universe or whatever power you believe in and work to save our environment and the elixir of life in abundance. Let's think big and "begin the world all over again."

Join Us

I'M NOT FAMOUS. I HAVE NO PLATFORM.
Very little social media presence. No orthodox creden-
tials for writing this pamphlet and expecting it to be read.
However, the truth is this pamphlet is not about me. All
of the facts came from the hard work of journalists and
scientists. I had the benefits of readers and editors on my
team. And now that the pamphlet is published (not for
profit), I'm hoping to attract people who will come to
believe that all Americans should understand the health
consequences of the Trump agenda before they vote.

We need Millennials and Gen Z-ers to read the pamphlet and then get their parents and grandparents to do
so as well. Donald Trump once said that he could walk
down Fifth Avenue, shoot someone, and not lose a vote.
He may be right, but it is my belief that when parents
and grandparents understand that his metaphorical gun
is aimed at their children and grandchildren, they will see
the urgency of voting him out of office.

We need the help of others. We need people to get the word out about the message in this pamphlet. We also have a two-page fact sheet, which can be downloaded from the sixonesevenbooks.com website. We're open to your ideas. We have three months to get as many voters as possible aware of how much damage President Trump has done—and will likely continue to do if re-elected—to the health of the inhabitants of the United States and the rest of the world as well.

Please join us.

Andrew Goldstein
andrew@sixonesevenbooks.com

Acknowledgments

———————

ALTHOUGH I HAVE WRITTEN THIS pamphlet in the spirit of the 18th-century patriots, I am struck by how extraordinary some of them were and how far short of extraordinary I am.

I don't say that with false modesty; I actually have a high opinion of myself. However, when I look over my careers in different endeavors, the main pattern I see is a person with a few talents needing the talents of others to succeed. This was definitely true in the custom-building world, where I had maybe four skills. Luckily, one of them was hiring and building a strong team. The same is true here. Composing this pamphlet, a feat numerous writers could knock off in a week or two—and something Alexander Hamilton could probably do in a few days—has taken me several months and more help than a 6,000-word pamphlet should require. I'd like to thank these helpers. Let me start with thanks to three M's: Mathias, Mila, and Michael Rosenfeld. Then there's Eliyanna

Kaiser, Joan Cocks, Peter Strauss, Eve Bridburg, my son Max, my daughter Lucy, my wife Pat, and my publishing partner, Michelle Toth. Some writers don't like editors changing their sentences. I love it. I love watching my writing get better. They all gave great advice. I particularly want to single out Scot Lehigh, a professional columnist, who copyedited the manuscript and offered excellent editorial comments. To paraphrase a lyric from Hamilton, "It's nice to have Lehigh on your side."

Lastly, I want to thank all of the journalists I have cited in this pamphlet as well as the many others who defend our democracy each day. In the face of a hostile President using a phony "fake news" label to discredit them, these journalists have been the front line in the battle to tell the real story of the Trump administration. Don't believe their partisan disparagers. The last few years have been a golden age of journalism.

Notes

---

i   Worldometer, Coronavirus Update

ii   *Ibid.*

iii   Richard Valdmanis, A tenth of U.S. veteran coal miners have black lung disease: NIOSH, *REUTERS*, July 19, 2018

iv   Alex Kasprak, Did President Trump Make It Legal to Dump Coal Mining Waste Into Streams? *Snopes*, February 6, 2017

v   Eliza Collins, Congress Passes Frist Rollback of Obama Environmental Rule, *USA TODAY*, Feb. 2, 2017

vi   David Cutler, PhD, Francesca Dominici, PhD, A Breath of Bad Air: Cost of the Trump Environmental Agenda May Lead to 80,000 Extra Deaths per Decade, *The JAMA Forum*, June 12, 2018

vii   Marianne Lavell, *Inside climate news*, April 19, 2017

viii   The Trump Environmental Record, *Environmental Protection Network*, April 22, 2020

ix   Exposure to Mercury: A Major Public Health Concern, *World Health Organization*

x   Mercury and Health, *World Health Organization*, March 31, 2017

xi   Brady Dennis and Juliet Eilperin EPA changing mercury pollution rule despite opposition from industry, activists *Washington Post*, 4/16/20

xii   Christine Ro, Coronavirus: Why some racial groups are more vulnerable, *BBC FUTURE*, April 20 2020

xiii   Chlorpyrifos, The toxic pesticide, harming our children and environment, *EARTHJUSTICE*

xiv   *Ibid.*

xv   Bess Levin, DOW CHEMICAL DONATES $1MILLION TO TRUMP, ASKS ADMINISTRATION TO IGNORE PESTICIDE STUDY, *Vanity Fair*, April 20, 2017

xvi   What is the Clean Power Plan? *National Resources Defense Council*, September, 29, 2017

xvii   Alex Formuzis, Trump's Scheme to Repeal Clean Power Plan Means More Kids with Asthma, More Early Deaths, Dirtier Air, *EWG Home*, August 21, 2018

xviii   Andrew Freedman and Chris Mooney, Earth's carbon dioxide levels hit record high, despite coronavirus-related emissions drop, *The Washington Post*, June 4, 2020

xix   Lisa Friedman, E.P.A. Plans to Get Thousands of Pollution Deaths Off the Books by Changing Its Math, *New York Times*, May 20, 2019

xx   The Trump Environmental Record, *Environmental Protection Network*, April 22, 2020

xxi   *Ibid.*

xxii   Juliet Eilperin and Brady Dennis, EPA to scale back federal rule restricting waste from coal-fired power plants, *The Washington Post*, November 3, 2019

xxiii   The Trump Environmental Record, *Environmental Protection Network*, April 22, 2020

xxiv   Coral Davenport, Trump Removes Control on Streams and Wetlands, *New York Times*, January 22, 2020

xxv   Impact of climate change on food production could cause over 500,000 extra deaths in 2050, *Science Daily*, source: *The Lancet*, March 2, 2016

xxvi   *David Suzuki Foundation*

xxvii   Alina Bradford, Effects of Global Warming, *LIVESCIENCE*, 8/12/2017

xxviii   Laura Tenenbaum, The World's Ocean Just Set The Record For Warmest Temperatures In Human History, *Forbes*, January 17, 2020

xxix   WMO confirms past 4 years were warmest on record, *WORLD METEOROLOGICAL ORGANIZATION* February 6, 2019

xxx   Michon Scott, Antarctica is colder than the Arctic, but it's still losing ice, *Climate.gov*, March 12, 2019

xxxi   Climate Change: How Do We Know? *NASA Global Climate Change*

xxxii   Rosemary Sullivant, NASA

xxxiii   Dr. James Wang and Dr. Bill Chameides, Global Warming's Increasingly Visible Impacts, *Environmental Defense Fund*

xxxiv   Alina Bradford, Effects of Global Warming, *LIVESCIENCE*, 8/12/2017

xxxv   Climate Change Adaptation: What Federal Agencies are Doing, *CENTER FOR CLIMATE AND ENERGY SOLUTIONS*

xxxvi   Helier Cheung, What does Trump actually believe on climate change, *BBC NEWS*, January 23, 2020

xxxvii   Climate Deregulation Tracker, Sabin Center for Climate Change Law

xxxviii   Coral Davenport, U.S. to Announce Rollback of Auto Pollution Rules, a Key Effort to Fight Climate Change, *New York Times,* March 30, 2020

xxxix   *Ibid.*

xl   Brad Plumer and Coral Davenport, Science is under attack: How Trump is sidelining Researchers and their work, *New York Times,* December 28, 2019

xli   Trump on climate change report: 'I don't believe it', *BBC NEWS*, November 26, 2018

www.ingramcontent.com/pod-product-compliance
Lightning Source LLC
Chambersburg PA
CBHW021339290326
41933CB00038B/982